# Soviet saboteur survival textbook (translated and edited)

* * *

# SOVIET SABOTEUR SURVIVAL TEXTBOOK
## (translated and edited)

Part 1

*Influence Of Physical-Geographical
Conditions On The Combat Capability
Of Reconnaissance Parties*

translated and edited
*by* **Andrew Senatas**

Andrew Senatas

PREFACE

## PREFACE

This text is the part of a real textbook written by one of the two most powerful Intelligence Communities in the USSR – the Main Intelligence Directorate (GRU) of the General Staff of the Armed Forces of the USSR (the USA equivalent would be the DIA (Defene Intelligence Agency)). It was titled: 'Ensuring the Combat Capabilities and Survival Abilities of Reconnaissance Parties' and was published in Moscow, in 1990.

At the time of publication and for some time after, this textbook was marked as 'Not for public use' and was used to help officers and NCOs of Soviet intelligence units to train reconnaissance troops.

The published text has been translated from Russian to English and includes a chapter entitled "INFLUENCE OF PHYSICAL-GEOGRAPHICAL CONDITIONS ON THE COMBAT CAPABILITY OF RECONNAISSANCE PARTIES". The chapter gives a brief description of the most extreme physical and geographical regions of the globe (the Arctic, Northern coniferous forest zone (taiga), deserts, jungles, and the Global Ocean) from the standpoint of survival factors. The structure of the text and illustrations are the same as in the original edition.

This book is the first in a series of publications that include interesting and useful chapters from the above textbook, which are applicable and that can be used not only by a narrow range of military specialists, but also by a wider range of readers, among which are tourists, fishermen, hunters, scouts, etc.

The specific feature of these text editions, written for the Soviet Intelligence Communities, is that they were the result of many years of experience of these organizations. In these publications, the results of specialized research done by various scientific organizations in the USSR and other countries are shown. In some chapters of the textbook, which are mostly devoted to the implementation of combat missions, references to foreign experience are described. It indicates that the authors of the textbook conducted a thorough study of potential enemies.

The text can sometimes seem dry and boring, though the reader must understand that he/she is dealing with a textbook, the task of which is to convey the right material to the students, as simply as possible. The manner of information presentation is often surprisingly simple and specific, which will undoubtedly be appreciated by the readers.

# CHAPTER 1.
## INFLUENCE OF PHYSICAL-GEOGRAPHICAL CONDITIONS ON THE COMBAT CAPABILITY OF RECONNAISSANCE PARTIES

## 1.1. Brief physical and geographical characteristics of the Arctic

The Arctic is an extensive area of the Northern Hemisphere with an area of about 25 million km$^2$ (9,65 million sq mi), 15 million km$^2$ (5,79 million sq mi) of which is water. Its southern border passes through the points where the average temperature in July does not exceed 10°C (50°F).

The Soviet Arctic is limited by the meridians 32°4'35" E in the West and 168°49'30" W in the East. The Soviet Arctic includes the sector of the Arctic Ocean including the marginal seas (the Barents Sea, the Kara Sea, the Laptev Sea, the East Siberian Sea, and the Chukchi Sea), numerous islands, archipelagos, and the coastal zone of continental Eurasia.

All year around, most of the surface of the Arctic Ocean and the marginal seas, is covered with a 2.5 m (8,2 ft) to 3 m (9,8 ft) thick layer of ice. It is a ice mass that is not frozen into immobility. The wind and the way they are formed make the ice fields continuously move. They move either slowly, barely covering a distance of 1 (0,62 mi) to 2 km (2,24 mi) per day, or fast, covering a distance of 40 (24,6 mi) to 45 km (28 mi) in just 24 hours. They can drift in a variety of directions, although there is a general line of drift, which is from the East to the West. As the ice fields move at different speeds, this unevenness of drift constantly leads to Arctic collisions. Then the ice either diverges, revealing smoldering black fractures in the ice, or they collide with great force, forming ice pilings. In the mid-ocean, the height of these ice cliffs do not usually exceed 3 (9,8 ft) to 4 meters (13,1 ft), but in the coastal areas, they can reach ten meters (33 ft) or more.

The main climatic feature of the Arctic is the length of time it has very low temperatures. The average annual air temperature in the Arctic never exceeds zero (32°F), and the average monthly temperature in winter falls to -40°C (-40°F). The minimum temperature of the Arctic Seas' coast reaches -50°C (-58°F). In the summer, the only place that the air temperature can be above 0°C (32°F) is in the South-Western part of the Kara Sea. This temperature lasts for 59 to 109 days (Cape Chelyuskin and Vaygach Island). In the Laptev Sea and the East Siberian Sea, positive temperatures last for up to 87 days, in the North-Western part of the Chukchi Sea, they last for around 84 days (from early June to September), and in the South for around 112 days (from early June to late September).

In summer, rain and fog take the place of the cold and windstorms. During the two summer months, there are up to 24 foggy days. In the Kara Sea, the East Siberian Sea and other seas of the Arctic Ocean, from 55 to 122 days a year are foggy. In autumn, the probability of a cloudy sky exceeds 80%. Frequent fogs in the Arctic make it difficult for anyone to astronomically determine their location, orientation, and movement.

The extreme severity of the Arctic climate combines low temperatures with strong winds (table 1.1-1.2). The higher the wind speed, the greater the cooling effect of negative temperatures. The strongest winds, which are accompanied by snowfalls, can be seen in wintertime. Winds with speeds over 20 m/s (66 ft/s) occur very often.

A characteristic feature of the Arctic, which determines the diversity of the climate, is the status of the light. If the lengths of night and day on the 66th parallel are quite even, then the farther

North you go, the longer the polar day in summer and the polar night in winter. At 70° N, the polar day lasts 7 days and the polar night lasts 59 days. At 90° N, they last 100 and 176 days, respectively. The status of the has a significant impact on all kinds of human activity in the Arctic. The polar night is particularly significant in this respect.

The flora of the Arctic is represented mainly by mosses and lichens of various species, but sometimes, herbaceous plants can also be found there. About 350 species of vascular plants belonging to 38 grass, cruciferous, and saxifrage families, are found in the archipelagos and islands. The autumn tundra abounds with mushrooms, most of which are edible. The farther to the North, the Arctic lands are more severe and lifeless, and for most of the year they are hidden under snow and ice.

The fauna of the Arctic, despite the harsh climatic conditions, is quite diverse. On the island and mainland tundra, numerous herds of deer and wolves can be found. Foxes and Arctic foxes are also inhabitants there. On the islands and archipelagos (Wrangel Island, Severnaya Zemlya), lives the 'master' of the Arctic, the polar bear, wandering in search of food up to the North Pole. Summer tundra is dotted with numerous traces of gnawing animals. However, the Arctic is especially rich in birds. There are more than 150 species of them. As winter sets in, most birds fly South, but some of them, such as the snow grouse, ptarmigan, and the snowy owl, stay in the Arctic to pass the winter. On the sea cliffs of Novaya Zemlya, Severnaya Zemlya, Wrangel Island, Preobrazheniya Island, and the Franz Josef Land seashore, colonies of birds represented by giant nesting seabirds (gulls, seagulls, Arctic loons, Brent geese, eider ducks and other geese) are found. In the seas and on the coast, some marine mammals such as eared seals, bearded seals, walruses, and Greenland seals are found. The coastal areas of the Arctic seas, as well as the freshwater bodies of the tundra and islands, are home to more than 150 species of fish (cod, char, haddock, perch, salmon, humpback salmon, and muksun), most of which can be used for food.

A feature of the fauna of the Arctic is the complete absence of reptiles. However, the insect world is very well represented. In the warm season, myriads of blood-sucking insects appear in the tundra. Mosquitoes, midges, black flies, and gadflies are its curse.

## Table 1.1 Wind chill index (european measures)

| Wind speed, m/s | Temperature, °C | | | | | | | |
|---|---|---|---|---|---|---|---|---|
| | 10 | 5 | 0 | -5 | -10 | -15 | -20 | -25 |
| 2-3 | 9 | 3 | -2 | -7 | -12 | -17,5 | -23 | -28 |
| 4-5 | 4 | -2 | -8 | -14 | -21 | -27 | -34 | -38 |
| 6-7 | 2 | -5 | -12 | -19 | -25,5 | -32 | -39 | -44 |
| 8-9 | 0 | -7 | -14 | -22 | -29 | -35,5 | -43 | -49 |
| 10 | -1 | -7,5 | -14,5 | -23 | -30,5 | -36,5 | -44,5 | -50,5 |
| 11-12 | -1,5 | -8 | -17 | -24 | -32 | -38 | -46 | -52 |
| 13-14 | -2 | -10 | -18 | -26 | -34 | -40 | -49 | -54 |
| 15-16 | -3 | -11 | -19 | -27 | -35 | -42 | -50,5 | -57 |
| 17-18 | -3,5 | -12 | -20 | -28 | -36 | -43 | -52 | -58 |
| | *Temperate zone* | | | | *Zone of increasing danger* | | | |

| Wind speed, m/s | Temperature, °C | | | | |
|---|---|---|---|---|---|
| | -30 | -35 | -40 | -45 | -50 |
| 2-3 | -33 | -38 | -44 | -49 | -54 |
| 4-5 | -44 | -51 | -57 | -63 | -69 |
| 6-7 | -51 | -58 | -65 | -72 | -80 |
| 8-9 | -56 | -64 | -71 | -78 | -85,5 |
| 10 | -58 | -65,5 | -74 | -80 | -88 |
| 11-12 | -60 | -67 | -75,5 | -83 | -90,5 |
| 13-14 | -63 | -70,5 | -78 | -87 | -94 |
| 15-16 | -64 | -73 | -81 | -89 | -97 |
| 17-18 | -68 | -74 | -82 | -90,5 | -99 |
| | *Dangerous zone* | | | | |

**Note:** At a speed of more than 18 m/s, any additional wind effect is quite negligible.
1 metre = 1,094 yard = 3,28 ft.
°F = °C*9/5+32

The islands of the Soviet sector of the Arctic cover an area of about 20 thousand $km^2$ (7,72 thousand sq mi). The largest of them in the Barents Sea are the archipelago of Franz Josef Land, Novaya Zemlya, Kolguev Island, and Vaygach Island, in the Kara

Sea – the archipelago of Severnaya Zemlya; in the Laptev sea – the Komsomolskaya Pravda Islands, the New Siberian Islands, in the East Siberian Sea – the De Long Islands, the Bear Islands, in the Chukchi Sea – Wrangel Island. The topography of the Arctic Islands is very diverse. In one area, it has a strongly pronounced mountainous character (Severnaya Zemlya, Novaya Zemlya, Wrangel Island), in another area, it has a hilly character (the New Siberian Islands), and on Kolguev, Vaygach, and Novaya Zemlya islands, there are mostly plains. Dome ice is quite widespread in the Arctic. It covers more than 42% of Severnaya Zemlya, 25% of Novaya Zemlya, and almost 90% of Franz Josef Land.

## Table 1.2 Wind chill index (american measures)

| Wind speed, ft/s | Temperature, °F | | | | | | | |
|---|---|---|---|---|---|---|---|---|
| | 50 | 41 | 32 | 23 | 14 | 5 | -4 | -13 |
| 7-10 | 48 | 37 | 28 | 19 | 10 | 1 | -9 | -18 |
| 13-16 | 39 | 28 | 18 | 7 | -6 | -17 | -29 | -36 |
| 20-23 | 36 | 23 | 10 | -2 | -14 | -26 | -38 | -47 |
| 26-30 | 32 | 19 | 7 | -8 | -20 | -32 | -45 | -56 |
| 33 | 30 | 19 | 6 | -9 | -23 | -34 | -48 | -59 |
| 36-39 | 29 | 18 | 1 | -11 | -26 | -36 | -51 | -62 |
| 43-46 | 28 | 14 | 0 | -15 | -29 | -40 | -56 | -65 |
| 49-52 | 27 | 12 | -2 | -17 | -31 | -44 | -59 | -71 |
| 56-59 | 26 | 10 | -4 | -18 | -33 | -45 | -62 | -72 |
| | Temperate zone | | | | Zone of increasing danger | | | |

| Wind speed, ft/s | Temperature, °F | | | | |
|---|---|---|---|---|---|
| | -22 | -31 | -40 | -49 | -58 |
| 7-10 | -27 | -36 | -47 | -56 | -65 |
| 13-16 | -47 | -60 | -71 | -81 | -92 |
| 20-23 | -60 | -72 | -85 | -98 | -112 |
| 26-30 | -69 | -83 | -96 | -108 | -122 |
| 33 | -72 | -86 | -101 | -112 | -126 |
| 36-39 | -76 | -89 | -104 | -117 | -131 |
| 43-46 | -81 | -95 | -108 | -125 | -137 |
| 49-52 | -83 | -99 | -114 | -128 | -143 |
| 56-59 | -90 | -101 | -116 | -131 | -146 |
| | Dangerous zone | | | | |

Along the Arctic coast, from the East to the West, there is a wide strip of tundra (almost 3 million km$^2$/1,16 million sq mi), which in some places reaches a depth of 600 km/373 mi. Its southern skirt (shrub tundra) is covered with coppices of dwarf birch and willow wood, the small stems of which are pressed to the ground. Northern tundra areas are Arctic deserts and semi-deserts, poor in vegetation and animal life. The soil of the tundra, frozen to a great depth, thaws only a few tens of centimeters in the warm season (0,5-2 ft). As a result, meltwater, not able to run off, is accumulated on the surface, forming countless swamps and streams.

The foreign Arctic includes the Northern regions of Alaska, Canada, Greenland, Jan Mayen Island, and Svalbard archipelago (Spitzbergen) together with the adjacent polar seas. The total area of the foreign Arctic is more than 17 million km$^2$ (6,56 million sq mi), 13 million km$^2$ (5 million sq mi) of which are the polar seas of the Arctic Ocean (Beaufort, Greenland, and Chukchi seas) and large bays with independent hydrological regimes (Baffin and Hudson bays).

\* \* \*

## 1.2. Humans living in conditions of autonomous existence in the Arctic

People can find themselves living an autonomous existence in the Arctic due to a variety of circumstances. However, whether these people are in the ice of the Arctic basin, or in the snow-covered tundra, cold becomes their main enemy. The fight against cold, with the impact of low temperatures on the body, is the most important problem for an autonomous existence in the Arctic. It is clothes that play an essential part in the prevention of cold injuries. The warmer they are, the longer people can withstand the polar cold.

There is a positive correlation of the time, during which the human body is warm enough, the ambient temperature and the heat insulation properties of clothing (fig. 1). The diagram shows that a person dressed in a summer jumpsuit, at a temperature of 0°C/32°F will be warm enough for no more than for half an hour (line A). A person wearing woolen underwear and a short coat with a quilted lining will be warm for the same amount of time at an open-air temperature of -30°C/-22°F (line B) or also warm for half an hour at a temperature of -50°C/-58°F if wearing a set of woolen underwear, a woolen sweater and a fur jacket with trousers. If one covers the jacket with a waterproof fabric and provides warm bedding, the person will begin to freeze after 55-60 minutes (line D). Even the warmest clothing can maintain a positive thermal balance at negative ambient temperatures for a very limited time. Sooner or later, heat loss will be greater than heat production, so the body will begin to cool. This process speeds up at a temperature of -12°C/10°F or below.

Clothing only conserves heat in the body for a limited time, and that is why scouts in distress should hurry to construct an emergency shelter. The best construction material in the Arctic is snow. It is easy to process, and it has excellent thermal insulation properties due to the high air content (up to 90%). Due to this property, the air temperature of snow shelters is usually 15 (59°F) to 20°C (68°F) higher than the surrounding open-air temperature. A facing made of snow bricks significantly warms any camping tent. With a 40 (1,3 ft) to 60 cm (2 ft) thick facing, one can keep the temperature in the tent 10 (50°F) to 15°C (59°F) above the surrounding open-air temperature, without using any heating devices.

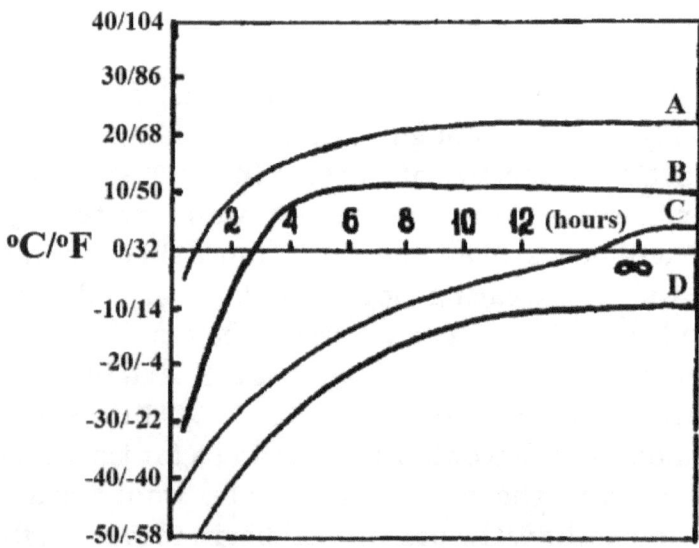

Fig. 1. The importance of the environment's temperature on the time the body will keep warm

°F = °C*9/5+32

The depth of snow cover in the Arctic is usually 25-90 cm (0,80-3 ft). However, the snow, moving under the influence of the wind, can form large drifts, which may sometimes be 1.5 to 2 m (5-7 ft) high. Their density is very high. In such a snowdrift, one can dig a snow trench using a military bayonet knife or any regular knife. To build a snow cave, one should create a tunnel in the snowdrift and expand its closed end to the desired size. If the snow is not so deep, to protect the cave from the wind, one can erect a half-meter (1,6 ft) wall made of small snow blocks placed transversely to the direction of the prevailing wind. To determine the direction, look at the location of small snowdrifts, to see the direction the wind has driven them.

It is thought that the most perfect shelter is the Eskimo snow shelter, called an "Igloo" (fig. 2). For its construction, it is necessary to find a flat area with dense and deep snow cover (at least 1 m/3,28 ft). Then, by means of a rope (sling rope), with a stake tied to both ends, one should draw a circle where the first row of snow bricks will be placed. The diameter of the circle should be chosen depending on the number of inhabitants: 2.4 m (8 ft) for one person, 2.7 m (9 ft) for two people, 3 m (10 ft) for three, and 3.6 m (12 ft) for four. Using a shovel (arm-saw, machete, bayonet-knife) one should move down wind and cut snow bricks of 45x60x10 cm (18x24x4 inches). To extract such a snow block, one should cut a gap of 5 cm (2 inches) on both sides. Then the knife is placed under the base and moved backwards and forwards with gentle movements. The trench formed after excavation of the blocks will serve as an entrance for the future shelter.

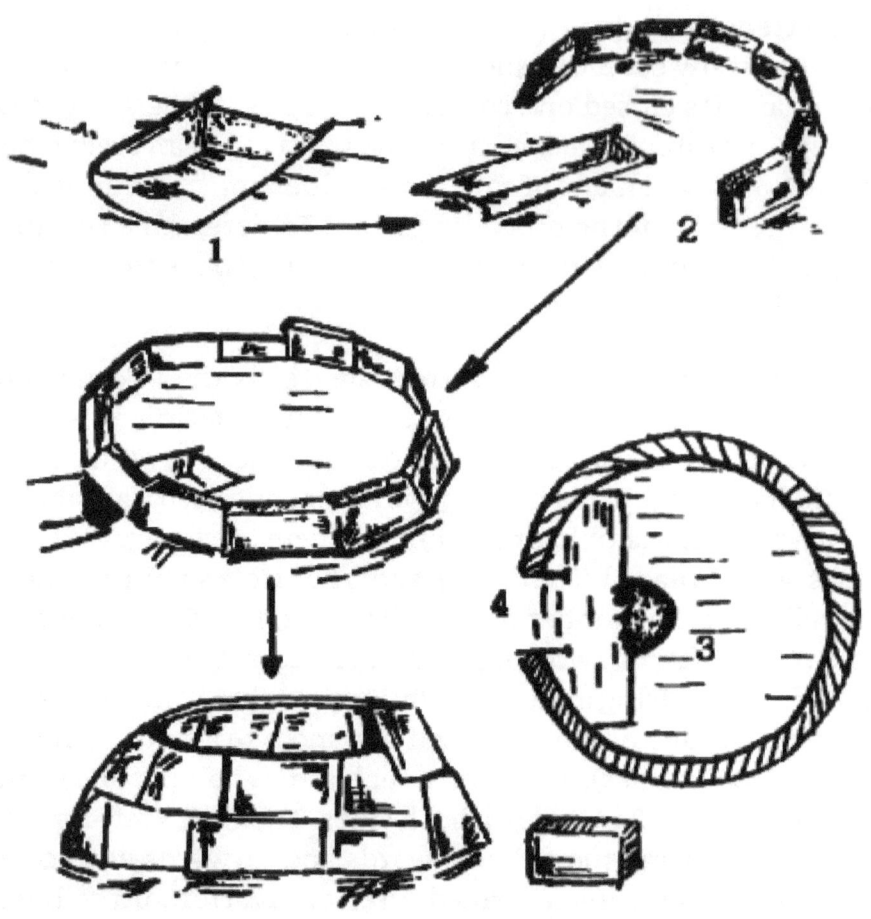

**Fig. 2. The order of construction of an "Igloo" snow shelter**

1 – a trench; 2 – blocks of the first row; 3 – bedding; 4 – the door

15 to 20 blocks are laid in the first row along the perimeter of a circle, with an inwards inclination of 20 to 25°. Then one should cut one of the blocks diagonally to its lower edge. In the hole formed, one should stack the first block of the second tier,

and then continue to lay blocks spirally. In this case, each block of the next row is placed under a larger slope than the previous one. When one finishes laying the walls, the holes between the blocks should be filled with snow. From the side of the trench, one should cut through the inlet in the wall of the igloo and make a sleeping ledge against the wall, out of blocks of snow, to a height of 60 to 70 cm (2 to 2,3 ft). The ledge should be covered with a tarpaulin or parachute fabric. Sometimes an inflatable boat (bottom up) can be put on it. To ensure ventilation, a small hole is cut in the top of the dome. An igloo can be erected in 1 to 2 hours.

An inflatable life raft may become another reliable shelter that does not require too much effort. Even with the most modest means of heating (two stearin candles) at open-air temperatures of -25°C (-13°F), the temperature inside the shelter can be raised from -20°C to +1°C (-4°F to 34°F). The temperature inside the raft can be even higher if it is further insulated with a layer of snow blocks.

For heating, cooking, melting snow, and boiling water a variety of means are used. Among them are stearin candles, fuel tablets, the fat of seals, walruses and polar bears, dwarf trees, peat turf, dry grass, fin (trunks and large branches of trees thrown ashore). Peat turf should be pre-cut into small briquettes and dried, and dry grass should be tied in bunches.

A fat lamp is the most convenient mean of heating a small shelter. Its design is quite simple. In the bottom of the can, one should punch a hole, through which a wick made of a piece of bandage, handkerchief or other tissue (previously moistened or rubbed with fat) is put. Pieces of fat are placed on the bottom, so fat, melting, drains down, keeping the flame alive. The air inflow is provided to the lamp by 3 to 4 holes punched on its side. A lamp of another type is made from a flat can, a first-aid kit box or simply a metal sheet bent at the edges. It is filled with fuel, in which 1/2 of the wick is immersed. A couple of such lamps can maintain a positive temperature in the shelter even with the most severe frost.

\* \* \*

## 2.1. Brief physical and geographical characteristics of the taiga zone

In the dictionary of Sergey Ozhegov, "taiga" is defined as "a wild, impassable forest in the North of Europe and Asia". Forests of North America and Canada can also fit into this group. From the geobotanical point of view, taiga is a zone of vast coniferous forests formed by one or many species of trees from the spruce group (sometimes mixed with some deciduous species). It stretches from Scandinavia to the shores of the Pacific Ocean, from the polar tundra to the Tien Shan Islands. High-boron Yenisei forests with their endless and impassable thickets, West Siberian swamps, Karelian landscapes with a dense network of lakes, short pure rivers, and moss moors are considered as taigas. Also among them are Pechora pine thickets with meadows, hills, and rocks, overgrown with lichen and crossed by turbulent, pure rivers, as well as the light cedar forests of Eastern Siberia and the dense wilds of Ussuriland with broad-leaved and subtropical trees.

The climate of the taiga is quite unique. A short hot summer, when the temperature often remains at 27 to 30°C (81 to 86°F), quickly changes into a hazy windy autumn. This is when drizzle or even hours-long pouring rains start. The average daily temperature is 0 to 10°C (32 to 50°F). Winter begins in November or December, then the temperature of the taiga decreases to 40 to 55 degrees below zero (-40 to 67°F).

The fauna of the taiga is very rich. Here one can find herds of deer and roe deer, noble moose and mighty wild boars, bears, wolves, wolverines, etc. The rodent family is represented by squirrels, flying squirrels, chipmunks, and hares. Numerous birds of various breeds can also be seen here. Among them are woodpeckers, crossbills, black grouse, hazel grouse, and wood grouse. Fish are bountiful in the taiga with graylings, pikes, and humpback salmon.

The real plague of the taiga is blood-sucking mosquitoes and midges. Myriads of them attack people and animals, blind them, and clutter up ears and noses. They mostly appear on sunny windless days, before rain, and at dusk. Even the smoke of fires and insect repellents cannot keep them away. Their bites itch unbearably, and the itching intensifies due to the scratching. However, the real hazard is posed by the ticks, carriers of encephalitis.

*　*　*

## 2.2. Humans living in conditions of autonomous existence in the taiga

There are many cases when people have gone to the taiga, and because they did not have enough experience and knowledge of the local conditions, quickly lost their way and, having lost their sense of direction, find themselves in distress.

A person who is lost in the taiga often gets terrified and confused. Eric Collier described this state in his novel Three Against the Wilderness (1971): "When one is badly lost in the deep woods and becoming more so all the time, it is only a short step from cool sanity to a state of feverish panic, and a madness of sorts besets you, so you now run, trip over wind-blown branches and fall headlong to the ground, you go on and on, indifferent to the direction, until finally physical and mental exhaustion is complete, and you lack either the will or the strength to go a step further."

How should you behave when lost in the woods? Having lost one's orientation, he/she must immediately stop moving and try to find the right way, using a compass or a variety of natural signs. If this is not possible, the best thing to do is to find a dry spot and arrange an encampment. This is not easy, especially in moss forests, where the ground is covered with a solid carpet of sphagnum, greedily absorbing water (500 parts of water per one part of dry matter). A canopy, a cabin or a dugout can serve as a temporary shelter. For convenience, for each member of the group, the area should be approximately 2 x 0.75 m (7x2,5 ft).

In the warm season, one only needs to construct the simplest canopy. For this purpose, two half-meter long (one arm thick) stakes, which have Y shaped notches on the upper end, are driven into the ground at a distance of 2 to 2.5 m (7x8 ft) from each other. A thick pole (carrier bar) is put across the notches. To it, at an angle of 45 to 60°, one should lean 4 to 5 poles, and then fix them with a rope (sling) or flexible branches. Aligned to the ground, 3 to 4 poles-rafters are tied. On the rafters, starting from the bottom, fir twigs with thick foliage or bark are stacked. They are stacked in a way that each subsequent layer covers the underlying layer to about halfway. One can make bedding from fir twigs or dry moss. The canopy has a ditch dug around it, so that, in case of rain, water would not leak into the shelter.

A cabin with two sloping surfaces is considered to be more convenient. It is built under the same principle, however the poles, in this case, are stacked on both sides of the carrier bar. The front part of the cabin serves as the entrance, and the back part is covered with one or two poles and fir twigs. Before one begins its construction, it is better to prepare the materials: bars, fir twigs, and bark. To obtain pieces of bark of the desired size, one should make deep vertical cuts in the trunk of a larch tree at a distance of 0.5 to 0.6 m (2x2 ft) from each other. Then, on the top and on the bottom, these strips are cut with large teeth of 10 to 12 cm (4-5 inches) in diameter. Then the bark is carefully peeled off with an ax or a knife. In winter, one can build a snow trench that will serve as a shelter. It is dug in the snow, at the foot of a large tree. The bottom of the trench is inlaid with several layers of fir twigs, and the top is covered with poles, tarpaulin or parachute fabric.

* * *

## 3.1. Brief physical and geographical characteristics of the desert

Deserts are known to be extremely arid regions of the globe, which are poor in water and vegetation. They occupy about one-fifth of the land surface. The desert climate is characterized by low rainfall, hot summers, high evaporation, and significant daily and annual air and soil temperature variations.

In Africa, the deserts occupy almost the entire Northern part of the continent (from 12 to 15° N to the shores of the Mediterranean Sea). The largest desert in South Africa, the Namibian Desert, stretches from the Atlantic coast to the Southeast, along with the Orange River valley. In the central part of the continent, there is a rocky semi-desert called the Kalahari.

In Asia, deserts almost completely cover the territory of the Arabian Peninsula (except for the mountainous areas), moving East to Iran, Baluchistan, Afghanistan, and the Indian desert called the Thar Desert. Deserts occupy the adjacent territories of Central and Eastern Asia.

In North America, the desert zone stretches along the Gulf of California, stretching from Lower California to Lower Colorado, and into the basin of the Great Salt Lake. In the central regions of Mexico, deserts are located between 20-30° N.

In Australia, deserts cover more than half of the continent with sand massifs.

The sizes of the deserts are completely different. The Sahara occupies 7 to 8 million $km^2$/2,7 to 3,1 million sq mi (nearly 25% of the total area of the African continent), the Kara Kum desert – about 350,000 $km^2$ (135,000 sq mi), and the Kyzyl-Kum – about 300,000 $km^2$ (116,000 sq mi). The Atacama Desert, stretching along the coast of South America, forms a thousand-kilometer strip, the width of which does not exceed 80 km (50 mi).

Desert climates are characterized by high air temperatures. The average shade temperature in summer exceeds 25°C (77°F) and often reaches 50°C (122°F). The intensity of direct solar radiation is extremely high due to the high transparency of the air. The annual total radiation in North Africa is 200 to 220 kcal/1290 to 1420 sq inch (near St. Petersburg it is 80 kcal/$cm^2$/516 sq inch). The sun heats the soil to 70 to 80°C (158 to 176°F). Metal objects become so hot that touching them can cause burns.

In the deserts of the tropical belt (the Sahara, the Atacama), there is no pronounced change of season during the year. However, the winter period is more favorable for human existence. In October to March (in the Northern Hemisphere) and in April to September (in the Southern), the average temperature does not exceed 10 to 12°C (50 to 54°F). The maximum night temperature rarely drops to 0°C (32°F). However, in December and February, on higher grounds, there are frosts with a decrease in temperature to -14°C (7°F). At sunrise, the temperature rapidly rises to 25 to 30°C (77 to 86°F).

The most important feature of the desert is that it is extremely poor in precipitation. During the year, there are no more than 100 to 200 mm (4 to 8 inches) of it, and in some areas of the Libyan and the Cuban deserts, its amount is almost zero. Rains in the desert are quite rare. However, these rare rains fall in the form of large downpours, accompanied by thunderstorms.

The air of deserts is very dry; its humidity in the afternoon ranges from 5% to 20%, and in the night, it increases up to 20 to 60%. Climatic conditions of deserts located in the coastal zone of the Atlantic Ocean and the Persian Gulf are more favorable. There the air humidity is very high (up to 80 to 90%) and changes of daily temperature are not so large. From time to time, dew falls, and fog appears.

The climate of the intertropical deserts (the Kara Kum, the Kyzyl-Kum, and the Gobi) differs from the deserts of the tropical zone. Winters there are especially severe and snowless. In the Gobi, for example, it lasts about six months (without thaws) with frosts up to 40°C (104°F). The climatic conditions of the summer period are the same as in the deserts of the tropical zone. Daytime shade temperature reaches 50°C (122°F). There is almost no precipitation. In the Kyzyl-Kum, their annual amount is only 5 cm (2 inches). Desert winds, as a rule, are hot, dry, and dusty. They are known for the constancy of direction, duration, and frequency of occurrence. The Sirocco, for example, blows in Africa from May to October, a few times per month. Winds often turn into a dust storm, raising clouds of sand. The air temperature at that time rises to 48 to 50°C (118 to 122°F). It is accompanied by a sharp drop in humidity.

One of the largest sand deserts is the famous Taklamakan, which stretches between the Pamirs, Tien Shan and Tibet for 1,200 km (746 mi) from West to East and 500 km (311 mi) from North to South. However, most deserts cannot be called a kingdom of sand, since sands occupy no more than 10 to 15% of their surface. The water part of the territory of the Kalahari (over 70% of the Sahara) is a so-called hamada – endless rocky plateaus, separated by valleys and depressions. The surface is dotted with silicon gravel, burnt by the sun. It may sometimes be covered with a black shiny skin, which is called a "desert tan" – a precipitate of iron and manganese salts, which dissolved from the groundwater that rose to the surface.

Another kind of desert terrain is a serir – a sandy plain covered with small gravel. A serir is also a smooth endless surface of destroyed rocks. A person who finds himself in a serir feels as if he/she is standing in the center of a flat plateau.

In the deserts of Central Asia and the Arabian Peninsula there are so-called takyrs – huge lifeless areas, stretching for many kilometers. They are covered with a smooth and solid clay layer, which has cracked into countless tetrahedral or hexagonal tiles. Takyrs are formed on the areas of former silty flood flows or accumulations of spring rainwater. However, most often deserts are complex, diverse crazy quilts of rocky and clay plateaus, hilly sands, endorheic basins, isolated mountain hills, salt marshes, and takyrs.

The hydrographic network of deserts is represented mainly by ephemeral corridors, in which water appears only in the rainy seasons and disappears after a few days or weeks. All the water forming these long drains is rainwater. Pouring rains that fall every 3-4 years and form powerful destructive flows, interrupting short but deep valleys with steep slopes, are called wadis. Wadis covers 200 to 250 kilometers (124 to 155 mi) along the Red Sea coast, spreading to the Nile valley. Wadis are also found on the Sinai. During the rain, a wall of water flows into such valleys, devouring everything in its path. Asian deserts are crossed by a dense network of creeks (dry corridors of temporary water sources). After heavy rainfalls, impetuous torrents often occur in creeks.

Lakes often contain salty or bitter-salty water that cannot be drunk. The main sources of fresh water in the deserts are groundwater and condensation water. Shallow pools of condensation water are formed due to the penetration of rare rains into the sand and condensation water from the atmosphere forming at the same time as a sharp decrease in air temperature. Freshwater levels in the Sahara, the deserts of Arabia and Iran are located at depths of between 3 to 5 (10 to 16 ft) and 20 to 30 m (66 to 98 ft). In the Central Asian deserts, their depth does not exceed 1.5 to 4 m (5 to 13 ft). To produce fresh water in these places, it is better to make a well. Most caravan tracks, highways, and paths, as a rule, runs through water sources. Distances between them are usually great (100 km/62 mi or more).

One of the features of a desert and the consequences on its climatic conditions is that it is poor in vegetation. Only areas of permanent water sources, oases, are rich in vegetation. However, there are only a few of them. Thus, oases occupy only 350 km$^2$ (135 sq mi) of millions of square kilometers (386 102 sq mi) of the Sahara.

The fauna of deserts is not very diverse. Mammals are represented by antelopes, gazelles, jackals, and hyenas. As for hoofed animals, one can see Persian gazelles and saigas, as for rodents – tarbagans, ground squirrels, jerboas, groundhogs, and sand-lances. Reptiles are represented by numerous lizards and snakes, many of which are poisonous. In the spring, there are lots of different birds near the water bodies. There are 74 species of birds in the Sahara. Among insects, there are more than 500 species of spiders, grasshoppers, ants, and mantises.

## 3.2. Humans living in conditions of autonomous existence in the desert

High atmospheric temperatures, intense solar radiation, strong winds, and lack of water sources create extremely unfavorable conditions for the autonomous existence of a person in the desert. It is known that in the desert, the human body receives a huge amount of heat (more than 300 kcal/h) from the outside.

Table 2.1 Probable term (days) of autonomous existence of a man in the desert depending on the ambient temperature and available water supplies (european measures)

| Maximum daytime shade temperature, °C | Water supply for 1 person, in liters | | | | | |
|---|---|---|---|---|---|---|
| | 0 | 1 | 2 | 4 | 10 | 20 |
| 1 | 2 | 3 | 4 | 5 | 6 | 7 |
| Staying under a tent | | | | | | |
| 49 | 2 | 2 | 2 | 2,5 | 3 | 4,5 |
| 43 | 3 | 3 | 3,5 | 4 | 5 | 7 |
| 38 | 5 | 5,5 | 6 | 7 | 9,5 | 12,5 |
| 32 | 7 | 8 | 9 | 10,5 | 15 | 20 |
| 27 | 9 | 10 | 11 | 13 | 19 | 29 |
| 21 | 10 | 11 | 12 | 14 | 20,5 | 32 |
| 16 | 10 | 11 | 12 | 14 | 21 | 32 |
| 10 | 10 | 11 | 12 | 14,5 | 21 | 32 |
| Movement at night | | | | | | |
| 49 | 1 | 2 | 2 | 2,5 | 3 | |
| 43 | 2 | 2 | 2,5 | 3 | 3,5 | |
| 38 | 3 | 3,5 | 3,5 | 4,5 | 5,5 | |
| 32 | 5 | 5,5 | 5,5 | 6,5 | 8 | |
| 27 | 7 | 7,5 | 8 | 9,5 | 11,5 | |
| 21 | 7,5 | 8 | 9 | 10,5 | 13,5 | |
| 16 | 8 | 8,5 | 9 | 11 | 14 | |
| 10 | 8 | 8,5 | 9 | 11 | 14 | |

The main problem faced by people who find themselves in the desert is to reduce the amount of external heat and the heat production of the body, as well as to increase heat transfer out from the body. It can be solved in three ways: with the construction of a solar shade, with the restriction of physical activity, and with the careful use of available water supplies (table 2.1-2.2).

Since the main part of the heat (up to 72%) comes from solar radiation, a simple solar shade can reduce its inflow by 72-114 kcal/h (fig. 3). Moreover, the shade saves a person from receiving 100

Andrew Senatas

kcal/h of solar radiation, which he/she would have received from the radiated heat given off by the sand.

Table 2.2 Probable term (days) of autonomous existence of a man in the desert depending on the ambient temperature and available water supplies (american measures)

| Maximum daytime shade temperature, °F | Water supply for 1 person, in gallons | | | | | |
|---|---|---|---|---|---|---|
| | 0,0 | 0,3 | 0,5 | 1,1 | 2,6 | 5,3 |
| 1 | 2 | 3 | 4 | 5 | 6 | 7 |
| Staying under a tent | | | | | | |
| 120 | 0,5 | 0,5 | 0,5 | 0,7 | 0,8 | 1,2 |
| 109 | 0,8 | 0,8 | 0,9 | 1,1 | 1,3 | 1,8 |
| 100 | 1,3 | 1,5 | 1,6 | 1,8 | 2,5 | 3,3 |
| 90 | 1,8 | 2,1 | 2,4 | 2,8 | 4,0 | 5,3 |
| 81 | 2,4 | 2,6 | 2,9 | 3,4 | 5,0 | 7,7 |
| 70 | 2,6 | 2,9 | 3,2 | 3,7 | 5,4 | 8,5 |
| 61 | 2,6 | 2,9 | 3,2 | 3,7 | 5,5 | 8,5 |
| 50 | 2,6 | 2,9 | 3,2 | 3,8 | 5,5 | 8,5 |
| Movement at night | | | | | | |
| 120 | 0,3 | 0,5 | 0,5 | 0,7 | 0,8 | |
| 109 | 0,5 | 0,5 | 0,7 | 0,8 | 0,9 | |
| 100 | 0,8 | 0,9 | 0,9 | 1,2 | 1,5 | |
| 90 | 1,3 | 1,5 | 1,5 | 1,7 | 2,1 | |
| 81 | 1,8 | 2,0 | 2,1 | 2,5 | 3,0 | |
| 70 | 2,0 | 2,1 | 2,4 | 2,8 | 3,6 | |
| 61 | 2,1 | 2,2 | 2,4 | 2,9 | 3,7 | |
| 50 | 2,1 | 2,2 | 2,4 | 2,9 | 3,7 | |

The required human behavior is always unambiguous and is aimed at reducing the heat production of the body. Each extra calorie of heat requires water consumption for its removal, and, therefore, will lead to dehydration. That is why any physical activity in the hot times of the day should be limited to a minimum. All work regarding the search for water and food should be carried out only at night, in the cool morning or evening.

In the desert, one cannot take off clothes, because they protect the skin from direct sunlight and greatly prevent the drying effect of hot air. At temperatures above 40°C (104°F), not only does the wind not cool the body but it also increases the wind borne heat supply. A nude person feels more comfortable than when he/she is dressed since the evaporation of sweat increases and the process of dehydration is significantly accelerated. The water loss of a nude person at an atmospheric temperature of 35-52°C (95-126°F) and a wind speed of 2.5 m/s (8,2 ft/s), which was 515 g/h (1,14 ld/h), is reduced, if wearing a burnous, to 342 grams/h (0,75 ld/h), though the clothes should be well ventilated.

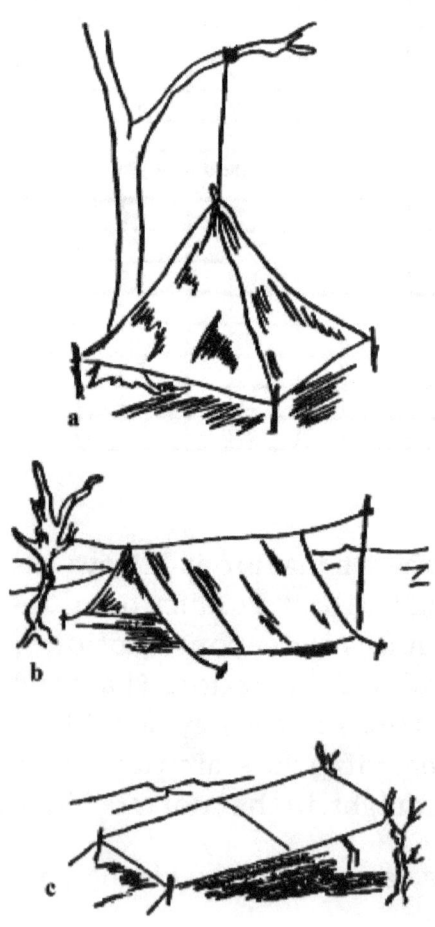

**Fig. 3. Some kinds of shelters in areas with hot climates.**
a – a canopy protecting from the rain and the sun;
b, c – a canopy for the desert areas.

Jungle covers vast areas of Equatorial Africa, Central and South America, the Greater Antilles, Madagascar, the South-West coast of India, as well as the Indochina and Malacca peninsulas, it also covers the Greater Sunda Isles, Philippine Islands, and New Guinea. Tropical forests occupy about 60% of Brazil and 40% of Vietnam. The jungle, (jangal) in Hindi and Maratha languages, stands for a forest or dense thickets. The characteristics of a jungle are similar to the features of a tropical zone. The average monthly temperature is 24 to 29°C (75 to 84°F), and their fluctuations during the year do not exceed 1 to 6°C (34 to 43°F).

## 4.1. Brief physical and geographical characteristics of the rainforest zone (a jungle)

The annual amount of solar radiation reaches 80 to 100 kcal/cm$^2$ (516 to 645 sq inch), which is almost twice as much as in the middle belt at latitudes of 40 to 60°. The air is saturated with water vapor; therefore, its relative humidity is extremely high – 80 to 90%. During the year, 1,500 to 2,000 mm (59 to 79 inches) of precipitation falls. However, in some spots like Debundscha (Sierra Leone) and Cherrapunji (India, Meghalaya) the amount reaches 10 to 12 thousand mm (394 to 472 inches).

Dense vegetation impedes the normal circulation of air masses, which is when the velocity of air is greater than 0.3 to 0.4 m/s (1 to 1.3 ft/s). High temperatures and humidity, as well as insufficient air circulation, can cause the formation of a dense radiation fog not only in nighttime but also in daytime. As a result of the putrefactive processes going on in the fallen leaves, the content of carbon dioxide (0.3 to 0.4%) significantly increases in the low layers of air. Therefore, it is almost 10 times higher than its normal content in the atmosphere. That is why a person, in the rainforest, often complains about the lack of oxygen.

The abundance and diversity of tropical flora has no match across the globe. For example, the flora of Myanmar is very rich. More than 30 thousand species (20% of the world's flora) can be found there. Favorable natural conditions contribute to the rapid development and growth of plants. Bamboo, for instance, grows at a rate of 22.9 cm/day (0,75 ft/day) for two months, and in some cases, the daily growth of its shoots reaches 67 cm (2,2 ft).

The evergreen vegetation of the jungle is multi-tiered. The first tier consists of single perennial trees up to 60 m (197 ft) high with a wide crown and smooth trunks without twigs. The second tier consists of trees up to 20 to 30 m (66 to 98 ft) high. The third tier is represented by 10 to 20 meter (33 to 66 ft) trees, mainly palms of different species. The fourth tier is a low underwood of bamboo, bushes, and ferns.

The main feature of a jungle is an extraordinary abundance of so-called off-tier plants – vines (the family of begonias, legumes, and Malpighian) and epiphytes (bromeliads, orchids), which intertwine, forming a solid green array.

There are two types of rainforests: primary and secondary. The primary rainforest, despite its many trees, vines and epiphytes, is quite passable. Dense thickets are found mainly on the banks of rivers, on the glades, in areas of forest clearing and fires. Secondary forests are characterized by giant trees that rise above the level of vegetation and are separated from each other at a great distance. Secondary rainforests are widespread in Central and South America, Central Africa, South-East Asia, the Philippines, New Guinea, and the Pacific Islands.

The fauna of the rainforests is rich. Here there are almost all kinds of large mammals (elephants, rhinos, hippos, buffalo, lions, tigers, cougars, panthers, and jaguars) and amphibians (crocodiles). Rainforest abounds with reptiles, among which there are a lot of species of poisonous snakes. The fauna of the jungle is considered to be a kind of "living pantry" of nature and, at the same time, a source of danger. The most dangerous and aggressive animals are the African buffalo, which attack people unexpectedly and for no apparent reason.

## 4.2. Humans living in conditions of autonomous existence in the jungle

A person who finds himself/herself in the jungle for the first time and does not have knowledge of the flora and fauna and the correct forms of behavior in these conditions, starts to doubt his/her abilities, expects danger, gets depressed and nervous. The uniqueness of the situation in combination with the high temperature and humidity affect the human mind. The pile of vegetation, which encircles him/her from all sides, constricts movement, and obscures visibility, ignites in a person the fear of an enclosed space. It is a condition, which is aggravated by the darkness, and filled with thousands of faint sounds. The condition manifests itself in inadequate mental reactions: retardation and, therefore, strong emotional arousal, which leads to taking hasty measures. As one gets used to the situation, this condition passes. Knowledge of the nature of the jungle and the methods of survival in it will contribute to successfully overcoming difficulties.

* * *

## 5. Brief physical-geographical characteristics of the Global Ocean

The surface of our planet is 70.8% covered with water. The Global Ocean consists of four oceans: The Pacific Ocean, the Atlantic Ocean, the Indian Ocean, and the Arctic Ocean. Geographers divided the Global Ocean into several zones, depending on their physical and geographical features.

Between 60 and 40° N, there is a temperate zone – a zone of cool waters and active cyclonic activity. In summer, the air temperature there rises to 22°C (72°F), almost coinciding with the water temperature. Weak westerly and southwesterly winds barely move the water surface. In this zone, the weather is usually cloudy, with drizzling rain and thick fog. In the winter months, the air temperature drops below zero (32°F). In the North of the Pacific Ocean, the air is cooled to -13°C (9°F). Winter brings the fervor of cyclonic activity, so storms are common in these parts.

The subtropical zone extends approximately between 40 to 50 and 30 to 40° N. The humid tropical air warms up to 24 to 28°C (75 to 82°F) in summer. However, surface waters remain relatively cold. Although the area is poor in precipitation, haze and fog are not uncommon. In winter, when the temperature difference between the water and the air causes increased convection processes, days with rain and snow are quite common. The weather is extremely unstable, and strong storms often take the place of sunny days.

The tropical zone, lying between 25 to 30 and 8° N, is characterized by high summer temperatures of water and air (25 to 27°C / 77 to 81°F). There is a little precipitation, and stable Eastern trade winds blow, without ceasing, all year round. In winter, the air temperature is reduced to 10 to 15°C (50 to 59°F). The probability of rain increases to 15 to 20%. From time to time, terrible hurricanes and typhoons bear down on the ocean. Then the white-caps get hidden in thick clouds that descend down to the water surface.

One can know if he/she has entered the equatorial zone, if there is a sharp weakening of the wind, increasing of clouds and frequent rain. The Equatorial zone is the hottest one in the ocean. Throughout the year, the mercury does not fall below 24°C (75°F) and may stay at the level of 30°C (86°F) for a long time. Annual temperature fluctuations are very small – only 0.5 to 1.5°C (33 to 35°F). Tiresome hot days are replaced by slack nights when the relative humidity rises to 85 to 95%. In the Equatorial regions of all three oceans, the temperature of the water is about a degree below the air temperature, which contributes to intense evaporation, the formation of cumulus clouds, frequent thunderstorms, and pouring rain. The duration of rainy weather in summer is 25 to 30% of the time.

The climatic conditions of the tropical and subtropical zones of the Southern Hemisphere are quite similar to the climatic conditions of the Northern Hemisphere. Its temperate zone is also called the "Roaring Forties." Storm areas, stretching along the meridian at 1,000 to 2,000 km (621 to 1243 mi), reach 55 to 58° S. There are frequent storms, raising waves to a height of 15 to 20 m (49 to 66 ft). The air temperature even in summer is about 0°C (32°F), and in winter it goes down to -10°C (14°F). Only in the Northern parts of the zone, does the temperature fluctuate to between 6 to 10°C (43 to 50°F) during the year. It is often raining and snowing there.

The largest current systems are anticyclonic and subtropical (low latitudes). They are extremely powerful and stable. They spread in the subtropics from one ocean coast to another, at a distance of 6 to 7 thousand km (3,7 to 4,4 thousand mi) in the Atlantic Ocean and 14 to 15 thousand km (8,7 to 9,3 thousand mi) in the Pacific Ocean. The main role in the formation of surface ocean currents belongs to the winds. There are Eastern trade winds that blow in the tropical zone all year round from East to West and form powerful equatorial currents (North and South). The speed of trade winds is 15 to 50 cm/s (0,5 to 1,6 ft/s). As they approach the equator, it increases to 100 (3,3 ft/s) and even 200 cm/s (6,6 ft/s).

In the Atlantic, the Northern trade current, penetrating the Gulf of Mexico, flows out of it at a speed of 9.35 km/h / 5.8 mi/h (Gulf Stream). When coming close to Chesapeake Bay, it carries 75 to 90 million m$^3$ (472 to 566 million bbl) of water per second. The most stable and rapid flows of the Global Ocean are the Gulf Stream and the Caribbean warm compensation currents (in the Atlantic Ocean), the Somali Current (in the Indian ocean), the Mindanao, the Kuroshio and the East Australian currents (in the Pacific Ocean). The flow rate is 25 to 50 cm/s (0,8 to 1,6 ft/s), sometimes 75 to 100 cm/s (2,5 to 3,3 ft/s).

The fauna of the ocean is extremely rich and diverse (more than 180 thousand species of animals). Areas of the cold and warm waters confluence are especially rich in animal life.

The flora of the ocean numbers about 15,000 species of algae. The most important edible algae are diatoms since no fish, shark, whale or human can survive without it. The color of the water tells volumes. The greenish color indicates the rapid development of plankton, while cobalt blue waves are beautiful but lifeless.

## CHAPTER 2. SURVIVAL FACTORS

The favorable outcome of autonomous existence depends on a lot of factors: the physical and psychological condition of the person, the supplies of water and food, the effectiveness of emergency equipment, etc.

The external environment and climatic conditions are very important for human life in conditions of autonomous existence. Environmental factors that affect a person are very diverse. Among them are temperature and humidity of the air, solar radiation, wind, etc.

The Arctic and the tropics, the mountains and the deserts, the taiga and the ocean – each of these natural areas is characterized by its own features, which influence the life of a person lost in a particular zone (rules of conduct, methods of obtaining water and food, construction of shelters, the nature of diseases and measures for their prevention). The harsher the conditions of the environment, the shorter the period of autonomous existence, the stricter the rules of conduct, and the higher the price to be paid for each mistake.

The favorable outcome of an autonomous existence depends largely on the psychophysiological qualities of the person (the will, resolution, discipline, wit, physical preparation, and endurance). However, having these important qualities may not be enough for survival. People have died of heat and thirst, unaware that just steps from them, there was a lifesaving source of water. They freeze in the tundra, unable to build a snow shelter, die of hunger in the forest, teeming with game, and become victims of poisonous animals, not knowing how to provide first aid when bitten. The formula for success in the fight against natural forces is his/her ability to survive. To survive means to apply all the acquired knowledge, experience, and ingenuity as well as using the available equipment and improvised means to protect himself/herself against the adverse effects of the environment, and to meet the needs of the body for water and food.

The fundamental premise of survival is that a person can maintain their health and their life in the harshest climatic conditions if he/she is able to take advantage of everything that the surrounding nature offers.

People who find themselves in the condition of having to lead an autonomous existence should perform a number of tasks, on which the preservation of their health and life depends.

Among them are:

- Protection from the adverse effects of environmental factors (high and low air temperatures, solar radiation, poisonous and predatory animals).

- Satisfying the body's need for food and water, and overcoming the stresses caused by the created emergency.

- First aid for victims.

- Orientation and positioning.

- Establishing communication and signaling.

## Table 4. Survival factors

| Survival motivation | | | | | |
|---|---|---|---|---|---|
| Positive factors | | | Negative factors | | |
| *Psychological* | *Physical* | *High training level* | *Psychological* | *Physical* | *Low training level* |
| high psychological training level | high physical training level | reasonableness of solutions | lack of will | low physical training level | ill-considered decisions |
| activity, resourcefulness, ingenuity | physical endurance | good knowledge of place and conditions | low psychological training level | low physical endurance | weak knowledge of place and conditions |
| discipline | | theoretical knowledge and practical skills | confusion, passivity<br>indiscipline | | weak theoretical knowledge and practical skills |

| Diseases | Stressors of survival | Physical and geographical characteristics of the area |
|---|---|---|
| parasitic diseases | stress from physical activity | temperature and humidity |
| thermal and cold lesions | fear | landscape |
| bites of poisonous animals and insects | thirst | rainfall |
| poisoning by animal and plant poisons | hunger | solar radiation |
| mental disorders | cold | flora |
| infectious diseases | overwork | fauna |
| injuries | loneliness | wind |
| exposure to military toxic substances | heat | water source |

When determining the environmental factors that adversely affect a person or group of people who find themselves in extreme conditions, the concept of "stress factors of survival" is used. Stress factors include pain, cold, heat, thirst, hunger, fatigue, despondency, and fear. This qualification is quite theoretical, however, it helps to systematize these factors, to consider them in interrelation with the external environment – a person in a condition of autonomous existence (group of tables 4).

Pain is a normal physiological reaction of the body that fulfills a protective function. A person, devoid of any pain sensitivity, is in serious danger because, in such a case, he/she cannot react to dangerous situations in a timely manner. On the other hand, pain, causing suffering, irritates, distracts and warns a person. However, strong, unbearable pain negatively affects his/her behavior and activities. At the same time, a person is able to cope even with very strong pain and overcome it, and by focusing on solving important, responsible tasks, he/she is able to forget about the pain.

Cold reduces physical activity and performance. Cold stress has an impact on the human mind. Not only muscles can freeze but also the brain and will can do so to, and without use of the brain any struggle is ill-fated. Therefore, in a low-temperature zone, for example, in the Arctic, human activity begins with measures to protect against the cold (construction of shelters, building a fire, and cooking hot food).

Heat. High environmental temperatures, especially direct solar radiation, causes significant changes in the human body, and sometimes in a relatively short time. Overheating of the body violates the function of organs/systems and weakens physical and mental activity. A lack of drinking water has the most dangerous effect on the body because, in this case, the body gets overheated and dehydrated. The construction of a sunshade, the restriction of physical activity, and the economical use of drinking water can greatly facilitate the situation of people in distress in the desert or the tropics.

Thirst is a signal of a lack of fluid in the body. If one cannot quench one's thirst in terms of an autonomous existence, it takes a hold of all his/her thoughts and desires. The main focus is on a single goal – to get rid of this painful feeling (with 5 to 6% dehydration, hoarseness appears, and 15 to 20% dehydration causes death. In some cases, depending on the physical costs and the state of the body, a person can lose up to 40% of their mass).

A set of sensations associated with the body's need for food is called hunger. It can be considered as a typical, albeit delayed stress reaction. It is a known fact that a person can do without food for a long time and still maintain efficiency. However, if one is hungry for a long time (especially along with the lack of water), his/her body weakens and reduces its resistance to the effects of cold and pain. Since the food supply is usually enough for a few days, the source of food should be the external environment. A person can obtain food through hunting, fishing, and collecting wild edible plants.

Fatigue is a kind of state of the human body that occurs after a long (sometimes short) exercise, or after mental stress. Fatigue is fraught with potential dangers since it dulls the will of a person, making him/her compliant to his/her own weaknesses. It prepares a person for the following psychological attitude: "This work is not urgent; it can be postponed until tomorrow." The consequences of this kind of attitude can be very serious. To avoid fatigue and quickly restore strength one can postpone physical activity and have a proper rest under any conditions.

Despondency is a mental state caused by loneliness, failure of conceived plans, unsuccessful attempts to establish communications, and unsuccessful attempts to get water and food. Its development is facilitated by non-employment, monotonous work, and the lack of a clear role. This state can be avoided by imposing duties and certain responsibilities on everyone, achieving their steady implementation, and setting specific feasible objectives.

<u>Fear</u> is the emotional reaction to danger and the most dangerous enemy for people who find themselves in conditions of autonomous existence. The reaction of a person to fear depends not only on the situation in which he/she finds himself/herself but also on his/her strong-willed qualities, organization, his/her assessment of the situation, and self-confidence.

For an untrained person, the external environment is a constant source of fear. Once in the forest, he/she is waiting intensely for the attack of a predatory animal. When afloat in the ocean, he/she is waiting with horror for the appearance of sharks. When on the polar ice, he/she is haunted by the fear that the ice would break, and in the desert, he/she would see poisonous snakes at every step. Although the feeling of fear is quite a natural reaction, if one does not cope with it, it will finally subjugate all his/her thoughts and actions. Fear turns any simple problem into a complex one and makes a complex problem unsolvable. "I do not believe that there are people who are strangers to fear... It is another matter when you overcome fear with spiritual power. I can agree with this, it is human nature," – says A. Zgeev, the veteran of the Great Patriotic War and the commander of a long-range bomber aircraft.

In a state of fear, a person loses the ability to control his/her actions and to make the right decisions. The state of fear increases the feeling of pain, the effects of cold, heat, hunger, and thirst. At the same time, fear, which is controlled and suppressed, can be a useful stimulant of human activity, forcing him/her to think faster and better, to act more intensely. It sharpens the perception of the senses, gives physical strength, turning the enemy into a kind of catalyst for energy and determination. Fear can not only reduce the chances of survival but also can significantly increase them.

The task of survival training is to achieve the maximum rapprochement between the ideal situation and the real one. The effectiveness of the training depends on the perception of the knowledge acquired in lectures, conversations, and class-room sessions. It is quite obvious that the moral, political, and psychological training of scouts plays a major role in the survival process. Without such daily purposeful training, it is difficult to expect success, since a person who does not have deep ideological convictions and a strong will, cannot resist difficulties and reso-lutely overcome them. In the moments of failure and danger, he/she is inclined to lose courage and give in to panic.

Regardless of the type of terrain where the scout is located, the chances of survival depend on the following factors:

- the desire to survive;

- the ability to apply existing knowledge, and strictly comply with the requirements of staying in a particular area;

- confidence in their knowledge of the area;

- judiciousness and leadership;

- disciplinary record and ability to act according to the plan;

- the ability to analyze any mistakes.

To survive means to solve three major problems.

Protection. It is necessary to think of shelter that would protect a person against cold, heat, winds, and overheating, depending on the terrain and weather conditions.

Water supply. Water, above all, is necessary for survival. At the earliest, one should set the daily norm. The reserve stock of water should be left as a last resort. One should take measures to find water sources.

<u>Food supply</u>. It is necessary to create a food ration. One should make sure that he/she has the required amount of water for cooking and consumption of food (when making the daily ration, one must remember that proteins require more water than carbohydrates for absorption).